Living With

Pancreatic Cancer

A Guide to Surviving and Thriving

By

Ellen D. Brandon

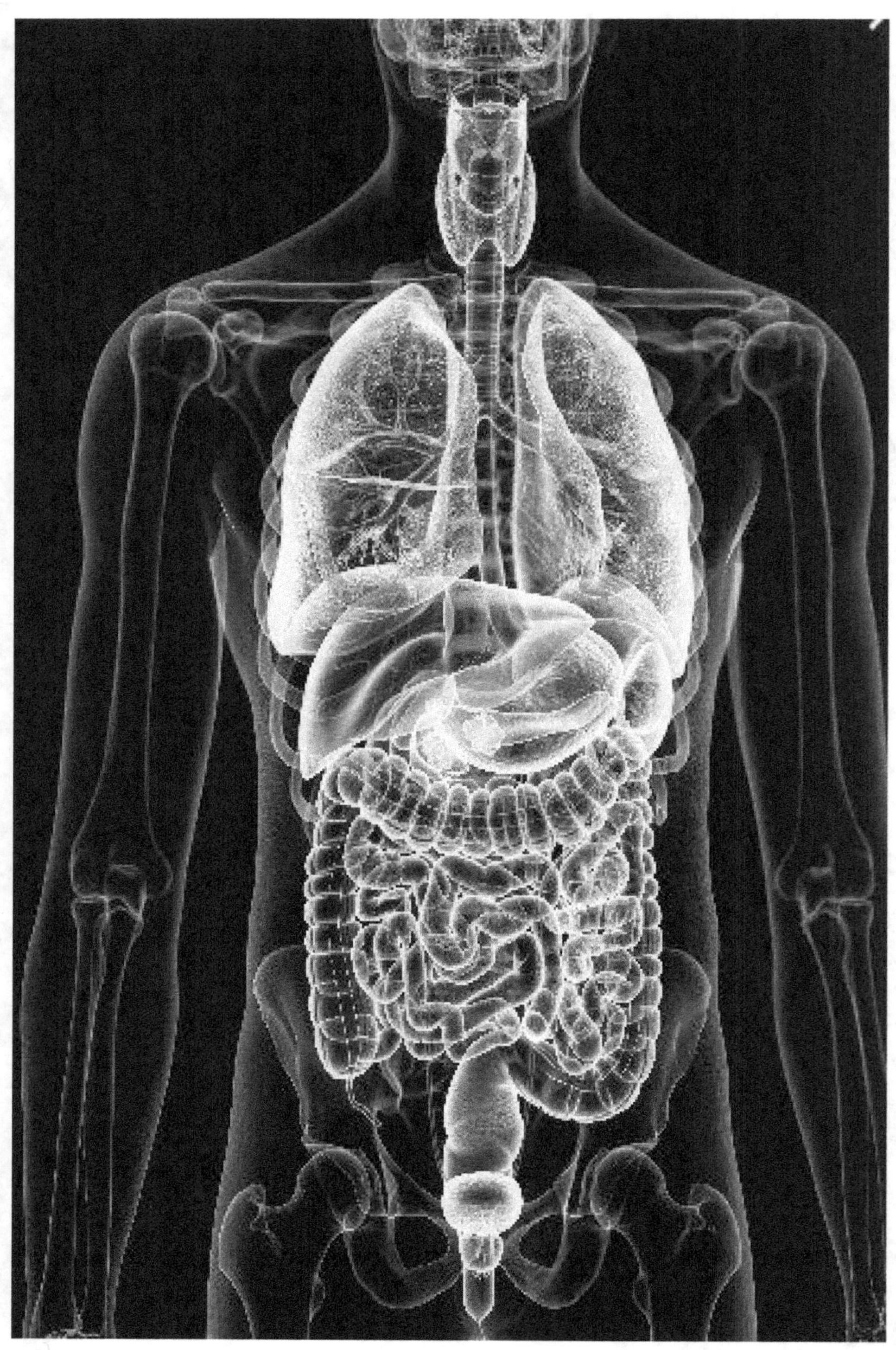

Copyright © [2023] Ellen D. Brandon

Table of Contents

<u>INTRODUCTION</u>

CHAPTER 4

Resources for Patients and Families

A. Financial and Insurance Assistance

B. Organizations and Support Groups

C. Other Resources

CONCLUSION

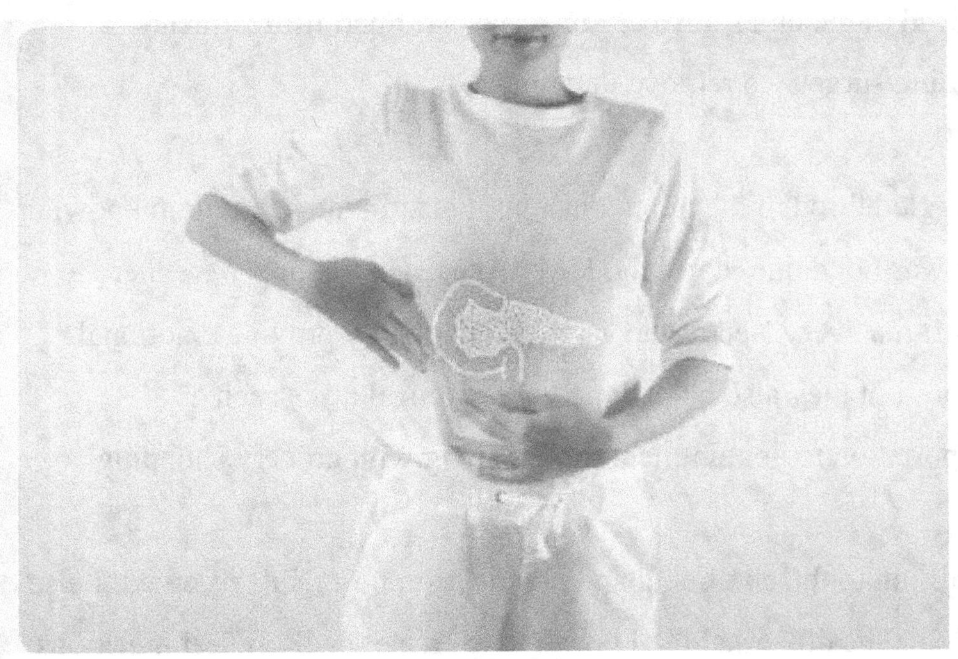

INTRODUCTION

I was a healthy and active woman until the day that I received an unexpected diagnosis. I was diagnosed with pancreatic cancer. It came as a complete shock. I was scared and overwhelmed by the news, but I refused to give up.

My oncologist gave me an aggressive treatment plan that included chemotherapy and radiation. I was determined to fight my cancer and I followed my doctor's advice. I underwent numerous treatments including surgery to remove the tumor.

I struggled through the treatments, but I also found strength in knowing that I was not alone in my fight. My friends and family were there to support me every step of the way. They not only provide emotional support, but they also helped me with practical tasks such as transportation to appointments and helping with grocery shopping.

In addition to the emotional and practical support that I received, I also developed healthier habits. I began to exercise regularly, eat nutritious meals, and meditate to reduce stress. These changes helped me to stay physically and mentally strong throughout my cancer journey.

My determination and the support of my loved ones paid off and I am now thriving and surviving with my cancer. I am grateful for the care and support that I have received and I am determined to continue to live life to the fullest.

Living with Pancreatic Cancer is an inspirational journey of hope and courage for those living with this debilitating disease. Written by an individual who has experienced it first-hand, this book provides a unique perspective on the challenges faced by pancreatic cancer patients and their families. This book provides insight into the physical, emotional, and spiritual struggles of living with a terminal illness while still maintaining a sense of hope and resilience. Featuring personal stories of courage and determination, Living with Pancreatic Cancer is an invaluable resource for anyone living with or affected by pancreatic cancer.

CHAPTER I

Overview of Pancreatic Cancer

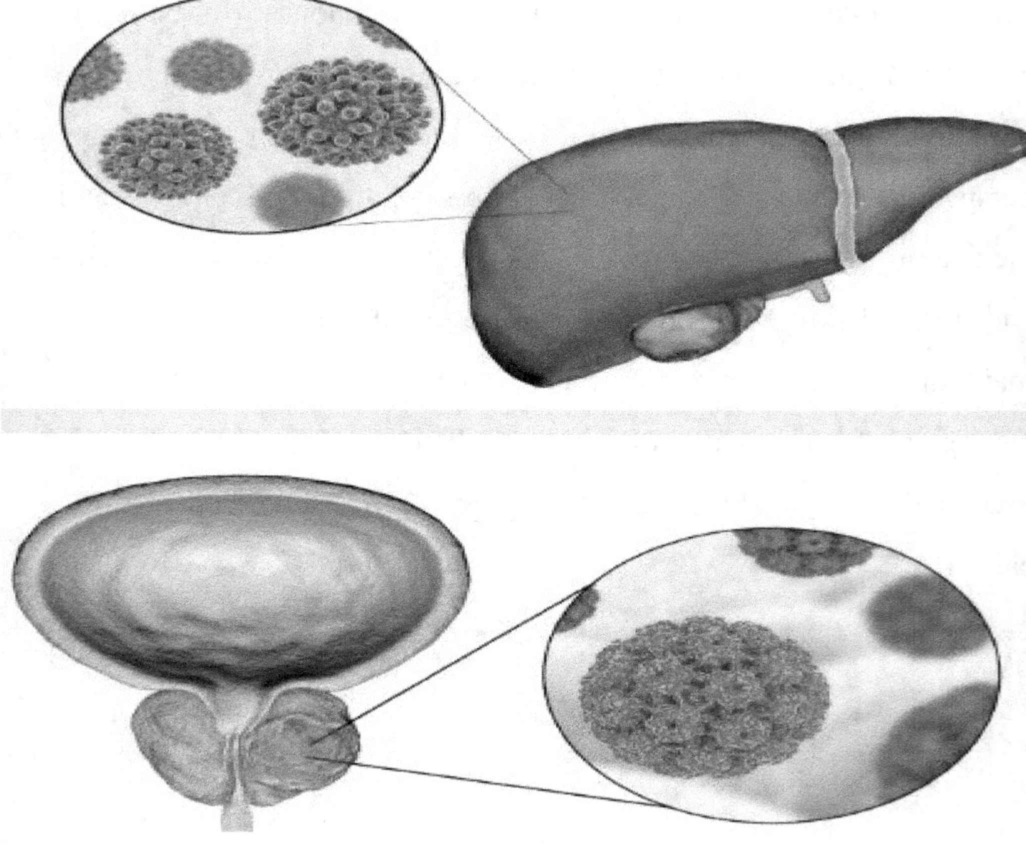

Pancreatic cancer is one of the deadliest forms of cancer, with an overall five-year survival rate of just 9%. It is a malignant tumor that starts in the pancreas, which is a small organ located behind the lower part of the stomach. The pancreas is responsible for producing enzymes and hormones that aid in digestion and regulate blood sugar levels.

Pancreatic cancer can spread quickly, and the most common type is adenocarcinoma, which starts in the glandular cells. Other types include pancreatic neuroendocrine tumors, which start in the hormone-producing cells; ampullary cancer, which begins in the ducts between the bile and pancreatic ducts; and cystic tumors, which form in the pancreas's lining.

The cause of pancreatic cancer is not fully known, but some risk factors include smoking, being overweight or obese, having diabetes, having a family history of pancreatic cancer, and being over the age of 65. Most cases are diagnosed in the late stages when the cancer has already spread to other organs.

Symptoms of pancreatic cancer can include abdominal pain, jaundice, weight loss, nausea and vomiting, dark urine, pale stools, and fatigue. Unfortunately, these symptoms can be caused by other conditions, so they can be difficult to diagnose.

Diagnosis is made through a variety of tests, including imaging tests such as CT scans and MRI scans, as well as blood tests and biopsies. Treatment options include surgery, chemotherapy, radiation, and targeted therapy. The type of treatment chosen depends on the size and stage of the cancer, as well as the patient's overall health.

Pancreatic cancer is a serious and life-threatening condition that requires prompt diagnosis and treatment. It is important to be aware of the risk factors and to seek medical attention if any suspicious symptoms appear. With early detection, treatment can be successful and survival rates can be improved.

A. Types of Pancreatic Cancer

1. Adenocarcinoma:

Adenocarcinoma is a type of cancer that originates from the glandular tissue in the body. This type of cancer is found in many organs, including the lungs, breasts, prostate, pancreas, colon, and stomach. Adenocarcinoma is the most common type of cancer in the United States and accounts for an estimated 40 percent of all cancers.

Adenocarcinoma is a malignancy that develops in the glandular tissue that forms the lining of the organs in the body. Glands are specialized cells that secrete substances such as hormones, digestive juices, and mucus. In adenocarcinoma, the cells in the glandular tissue become cancerous and grow uncontrollably. This type of cancer typically grows slowly and can spread to other parts of the body, including the lymph nodes, bones, and liver.

Adenocarcinoma is usually diagnosed through a combination of imaging tests and biopsies. Imaging tests such as CT scans, MRI scans, and PET scans are often used to detect the presence of a tumor. Biopsies are used to take a sample of the tumor to determine its type and whether it is malignant.

Adenocarcinoma is usually treated with surgery, radiation, and chemotherapy. Surgery is usually the first line of treatment and is used to remove the tumor and any nearby lymph nodes. Radiation and chemotherapy are used to kill any remaining cancer cells and reduce the risk of cancer spreading to other parts of the body.

Adenocarcinoma is a serious form of cancer that can be life-threatening if not treated effectively. It is important to seek prompt medical attention if you have any symptoms that may indicate adenocarcinoma. Common symptoms include changes in bowel habits, abdominal pain, blood in stool, and unexplained weight loss.

Examples of adenocarcinoma include prostate cancer, lung cancer, pancreatic cancer, and colon cancer. These types of cancer are typically diagnosed through imaging tests and biopsies.Surgery, radiation, and chemotherapy are treatments involved.

Adenocarcinoma can be a serious and life-threatening form of cancer, but with early detection and treatment, the prognosis can be good. It is important to seek prompt medical attention if you have any symptoms that may indicate adenocarcinoma.

2. Neuroendocrine tumors (NETs):

Neuroendocrine tumors (NETs) are a type of cancer that develops in the neuroendocrine cells of the body. These cells, which are found in organs such as the pancreas, lungs, and gastrointestinal tract, produce hormones and other substances that are important for normal body functioning. NETs are very rare, accounting for less than 1% of all cancers.

NETs can be divided into two main groups: functioning and non-functioning. Functioning NETs produce hormones that can result in a variety of symptoms, including flushing, diarrhea, weight loss, and abdominal pain. Non-functioning NETs do not produce any hormones and are usually found incidentally during medical imaging tests.

NETs can be further classified based on the type of cells from which they originate. These include pancreatic NETs, which originate in the pancreas; bronchial NETs, which originate in the lungs; and gastrointestinal NETs, which originate in the gastrointestinal tract.

NETs are typically slow growing and can sometimes be present in the body for years before they are diagnosed. Diagnosis of NETs usually involves the use of imaging tests such as CT scans, MRI scans, and PET scans. In addition, biopsies of the tissue can also be used to confirm a diagnosis.

Treatment of NETs depends on the location and size of the tumor, as well as the patient's overall health. Surgery is the most common form of treatment and is used to remove the tumor. In some cases, radiation and/or chemotherapy may be used to shrink the tumor or stop its progression. In some cases, medication may be used to reduce the symptoms associated with NETs.

NETs can be a serious and life-threatening condition, but with early detection and proper treatment, the prognosis for patients is usually good. However, it is important to monitor for recurrence of the tumor, as this may require additional treatment.

In conclusion, NETs are a rare type of cancer that can produce a variety of symptoms, depending on the type and location of the tumor. Diagnosis of NETs usually involves the use of imaging tests and biopsies, and treatment usually involves surgery, radiation, and/or chemotherapy. If detected early and treated appropriately, NETs can often be managed successfully, leading to a good prognosis for patients.

3. Pancreatoblastoma:

Pancreatoblastoma is a rare type of cancer that affects the pancreas. It is most common in children and is classified as an embryonal tumor, meaning it is formed from cells that have not yet fully developed. Pancreatoblastoma is a malignant tumor, meaning it is cancerous and can spread to other parts of the body.

The pancreas is a gland located behind the stomach and is responsible for producing enzymes that help break down food. It also produces hormones, such as insulin, which helps regulate blood sugar levels. When a pancreatoblastoma forms, it usually grows in the tail of the pancreas.

Pancreatoblastomas are typically discovered through medical imaging, such as a CT or MRI scan. Symptoms of pancreatoblastoma can vary depending on the size, location, and spread of the tumor. Common symptoms include abdominal pain, jaundice, weight loss, and blood clots. These are often caused by the tumor pressing on other organs and structures in the abdomen.

Treatment for pancreatoblastoma usually involves surgery to remove the tumor, as well as chemotherapy and/or radiation therapy to destroy any remaining cancer cells. In some cases, doctors may also recommend a liver transplant if the pancreatoblastoma has spread to the liver.

Pancreatoblastoma is a rare type of cancer that can be difficult to diagnose and treat. However, with early detection and treatment, the prognosis is generally good. Parents need to be aware of the symptoms of pancreatoblastoma so that they can seek medical attention if their child is exhibiting any of them.

In conclusion, pancreatoblastoma is a rare type of cancer that affects the pancreas and is most common in children. It is typically diagnosed

through medical imaging and can have a range of symptoms depending on the size and location of the tumor.
Treatment usually involves surgery, chemotherapy, and/or radiation, and the prognosis is generally good with early detection and treatment.

4. Solid pseudopapillary tumors (SPTs):
Solid pseudopapillary tumors (SPT) are rare, non-malignant neoplasms that typically arise from the pancreas. They can also occur in other organs such as the ovaries, ovaries, and the mesentery. The tumors are composed of solid and cystic areas as well as a pseudopapillary architecture. SPTs are usually benign but can be locally aggressive and metastasize, usually to the liver.

The most common type of SPT is the pancreatic variety, which affects women more often than men and usually occurs in young adults between the ages of 10 and 25. It is characterized by a large mass in the pancreas with a cystic component, solid pseudopapillary architecture, and a capsule. The tumors are composed of a mixture of epithelial, spindle, and stromal cells and can be associated with a variety of cystic spaces.

The clinical presentation of SPT is variable, but the most common symptoms are abdominal pain, nausea, vomiting, and jaundice. Imaging studies, such as MRI, CT scan, and ultrasound, can help diagnose the tumor and its extent. In some cases, a biopsy may be necessary for definitive diagnosis.

Treatment of SPT usually involves surgical resection, which is typically curative. However, chemotherapy and radiotherapy may be used if the tumor is more advanced or if the tumor is not completely resected.

The prognosis for SPT is generally good, with a 5-year survival rate of 80-90%. However, the risk of recurrence is higher in younger patients, and the risk of metastasis increases with the size and stage of the tumor. Therefore, regular follow-up with imaging and laboratory tests is recommended to monitor for recurrence or metastasis.

In conclusion, solid pseudopapillary tumors (SPT) are rare, non-malignant neoplasms that typically arise from the pancreas. They are usually benign but can be locally aggressive and metastasize. The clinical presentation, diagnosis, and treatment of SPT are variable but typically involve surgical resection. The prognosis for SPT is generally good, but regular follow-up is recommended to monitor for recurrence or metastasis.

5. Acinar cell carcinoma:

Acinar cell carcinoma (ACC) is a rare type of cancer that originates in acinar cells, or the cells that make up the glands that produce and secrete hormones and other substances. It is a malignant tumor and is most commonly seen in the pancreas, although it can also occur in other organs. ACC is a very aggressive type of cancer with a poor prognosis.

ACC is caused by mutations in the genes that control the growth and development of acinar cells. These mutations can cause the cells to divide and multiply abnormally, resulting in a tumor. The exact cause of these mutations is not known, but it is believed to be linked to certain environmental factors, such as exposure to certain chemicals or radiation.

The most common symptom of ACC is abdominal pain. Other symptoms include jaundice, weight loss, fatigue, and nausea. A diagnosis of ACC is usually made after a physical exam, imaging tests (such as CT and MRI scans), and a biopsy of the tumor.

Treatment for ACC typically involves a combination of surgery, chemotherapy, and radiation. Surgery is the most common treatment for ACC and may involve the removal of the tumor, as well as surrounding tissue and organs, depending on the size and location of the tumor. Chemotherapy and radiation may be used to shrink the tumor before or after surgery or to treat any remaining cancer cells after surgery.

ACC is a very aggressive type of cancer, and the prognosis is usually poor. The average five-year survival rate for ACC is around 10%, although this may vary depending on the size and location of the tumor, as well as the patient's overall health and response to treatment.

Due to the rarity of ACC, there is not much information available about the long-term effects of the disease. However, it is known that ACC can spread to other organs, and it is important to remain vigilant with regular checkups and follow-up care to monitor any possible changes in the tumor and the patient's overall health.

ACC is a serious and life-threatening illness, and it is important to be aware of the signs and symptoms and to seek medical attention if any suspicious symptoms arise. Early diagnosis and treatment can greatly improve the chances of survival and a better quality of life.

6. Cystic neoplasms of the pancreas:

Cystic neoplasms of the pancreas are abnormal growths or tumors that form in the pancreas and contain a fluid-filled sac or cyst. These growths can be harmless, meaning noncancerous, or threatening, meaning dangerous. Benign cystic neoplasms of the pancreas include pseudocysts, serous cystadenomas, mucinous cystic tumors, intraductal papillary mucinous neoplasms, and solid pseudopapillary tumors. Malignant cystic neoplasms of the pancreas include cystic neuroendocrine tumors and mucinous cystic neoplasms.

Pseudocysts are the most common type of benign cystic neoplasm of the pancreas. They are fluid-filled sacs that are usually caused by trauma or inflammation of the pancreas. They do not contain cells, so they are not tumors. Pseudocysts do not cause any symptoms and can resolve on their own.

Serous cystadenomas are the second most common type of benign cystic neoplasm of the pancreas. They are typically filled with a clear, watery fluid. They can range in size from small to large, and they do not usually cause any symptoms.

Mucinous cystic tumors are rare benign cystic neoplasms of the pancreas. They are typically filled with a thick, mucus-like fluid. They may cause abdominal pain or a feeling of fullness.

Intraductal papillary mucinous neoplasms are benign cystic neoplasms of the pancreas that form in the ducts of the pancreas. They can range in size from small to large and may cause abdominal pain or a feeling of fullness.

Solid pseudopapillary tumors are rare, benign cystic tumors of the pancreas. They are made up of a mixture of solid and cystic components. They may cause abdominal pain or a feeling of fullness.

Cystic neuroendocrine tumors are malignant cystic neoplasms of the pancreas. They are typically filled with clear, watery fluid and may cause abdominal pain, nausea, and vomiting.

Mucinous cystic neoplasms are malignant cystic neoplasms of the pancreas. They are typically filled with thick, mucus-like fluid and may cause abdominal pain, nausea, and vomiting.

In conclusion, cystic neoplasms of the pancreas are abnormal growths or tumors that form in the pancreas and contain a fluid-filled sac or cyst. These growths can be harmless, meaning noncancerous, or threatening, meaning dangerous. Benign cystic neoplasms of the pancreas include pseudocysts, serous cystadenomas, mucinous cystic tumors, intraductal papillary mucinous neoplasms, and solid pseudopapillary tumors. Malignant cystic neoplasms of the pancreas include cystic neuroendocrine tumors and mucinous cystic neoplasms. Treatment of cystic neoplasms of the pancreas depends on the type and stage of the tumor and can include surgery, chemotherapy, or radiation therapy.

7. Intraductal papillary mucinous neoplasm (IPMN): This is a type of cystic tumor that develops in the pancreas, a gland that produces enzymes and hormones to help digest food and regulate blood sugar levels. IPMNs are most commonly found in the main ducts of the pancreas but can occur in the side (branch) ducts as well. These tumors are typically benign, or noncancerous, and can grow slowly over many years.

IPMNs are divided into three categories based on their appearance and behavior.

The first type is the noninvasive IPMN (or main duct IPMN). This type is typically found in the main duct of the pancreas and usually does not spread to other parts of the body. These tumors can grow slowly over time and often have no symptoms. However, they may obstruct the pancreatic duct, leading to abdominal pain and jaundice.

The second type is the invasive IPMN (or branch duct IPMN). This type is typically found in the side (branch) ducts of the pancreas and can spread to other parts of the body, such as the liver or lungs. These tumors tend to grow more rapidly than noninvasive IPMNs and can cause abdominal pain, jaundice, and weight loss.

The third type is malignant IPMN or pancreatic cancer. This type is the most serious, as it can spread to other parts of the body and can be difficult to treat. Symptoms of this type of IPMN include abdominal pain, jaundice, and weight loss.

Most IPMNs can be treated with surgery to remove the tumor. Depending on the type of tumor, other treatments may be necessary. For example, if the tumor is invasive or malignant, chemotherapy or radiation may be used to reduce the risk of recurrence or spread.

IPMNs are relatively rare, with an estimated incidence in the United States of 1 in 100,000 people. Risk factors for developing IPMN include age over 50, family history of pancreatic cancer, and certain genetic mutations.

In conclusion, IPMN is a type of cystic tumor that develops in the pancreas. It is usually benign but can be invasive or malignant. IPMN can obstruct the pancreatic duct, leading to abdominal pain and jaundice. Treatment typically involves surgery but may include chemotherapy or radiation if the tumor is invasive or malignant. Risk factors for developing IPMN include age over 50, family history of pancreatic cancer, and certain genetic mutations.

8. Mucinous cystic neoplasm (MCN);

Mucinous Cystic Neoplasm (MCN) is a type of tumor that is made up of mucin-filled cysts. It is a relatively rare type of tumor, but one that can have serious implications depending on the type and location of the tumor. MCN can occur in various organs such as the pancreas and ovaries, but is most commonly found in the gallbladder.

Mucinous Cystic Neoplasms of the gallbladder, also referred to as MCGN, typically have a slow-growing nature and may not cause any symptoms. However, as the tumor grows it can cause blockages in the gallbladder, creating a risk of gallbladder rupture or gallstone formation. MCN may also cause abdominal pain, nausea, and vomiting.

The diagnosis of MCN is typically done through imaging studies such as an ultrasound, CT scan, or MRI. These imaging studies can be used to measure the size and shape of the tumor, as well as to determine if there are any signs of blockage or gallstone formation.

In order to determine whether the tumor is cancerous or benign, a biopsy may also be performed.

Treatment for MCN typically involves surgical removal of the tumor, as well as any associated blockages or gallstones. This may be done through a laparoscopic or open procedure, depending on the size and location of the tumor. In certain cases, chemotherapy or radiation therapy may be recommended to reduce the size of the tumor before surgery.

For benign cases of MCN, a watchful waiting approach may be taken, with regular follow-up imaging studies to monitor for any changes in the tumor.

For malignant cases, a more aggressive approach may be taken, as the goal is to remove the tumor and any associated blockages before the tumor can spread.

MCN is a rare type of tumor, but it is important to be aware of the symptoms and to seek medical attention if any are present. Early diagnosis and treatment can help to reduce the risk of complications and improve the outlook for affected individuals.

9. Metastatic tumors of the pancreas

Metastatic tumors of the pancreas are tumors that have spread from another part of the body to the pancreas. These tumors are also called secondary tumors or metastases, and they can originate from any type of cancer. The most common cancers that spread to the pancreas are lung cancer, breast cancer, and colorectal cancer, but other types of cancer can also spread to the pancreas.

Metastatic tumors of the pancreas can be difficult to diagnose, as they may not cause any symptoms in the early stages. When symptoms do occur, they may include pain in the upper abdomen, nausea, jaundice, weight loss, and fatigue. Imaging tests, such as CT scans or MRI scans, may be used to detect metastatic tumors of the pancreas.

Once a metastatic tumor of the pancreas is detected, it is important to determine the type of cancer that it originated from to determine the best treatment options. Treatment for metastatic tumors of the pancreas may include chemotherapy or radiation therapy, or a combination of both. Surgery may also be recommended to remove the tumor, although this is not always possible due to the location of the tumor in the pancreas.

In some cases, surgery may be combined with other treatments, such as targeted therapies or immunotherapies, to reduce the size of the tumor or to prevent it from spreading further. These treatments can help to slow the progression of cancer and improve the patient's quality of life.

Metastatic tumors of the pancreas can be difficult to treat and may be life-threatening if left untreated. It is important to seek medical attention as soon as possible if you experience any symptoms associated with metastatic tumors of the pancreas. Early diagnosis and treatment can help to improve the prognosis and may even result in a cure.

B. Staging Pancreatic Cancer

Staging pancreatic cancer is an important step in determining the best course of treatment and prognosis for a patient. The organizing framework used to decide pancreatic disease is the American Joint Council on Malignant growth (AJCC) TNM framework. This system classifies tumors based on their size, the extent of local spread, and the presence of distant metastases.

The T stage of pancreatic cancer refers to the size of the tumor. T1 tumors are small and confined to the pancreas. T2 tumors are larger than T1 but still confined to the pancreas. T3 tumors have extended beyond the pancreas and may have spread to nearby organs or tissues. T4 tumors have spread to distant organs or tissues.

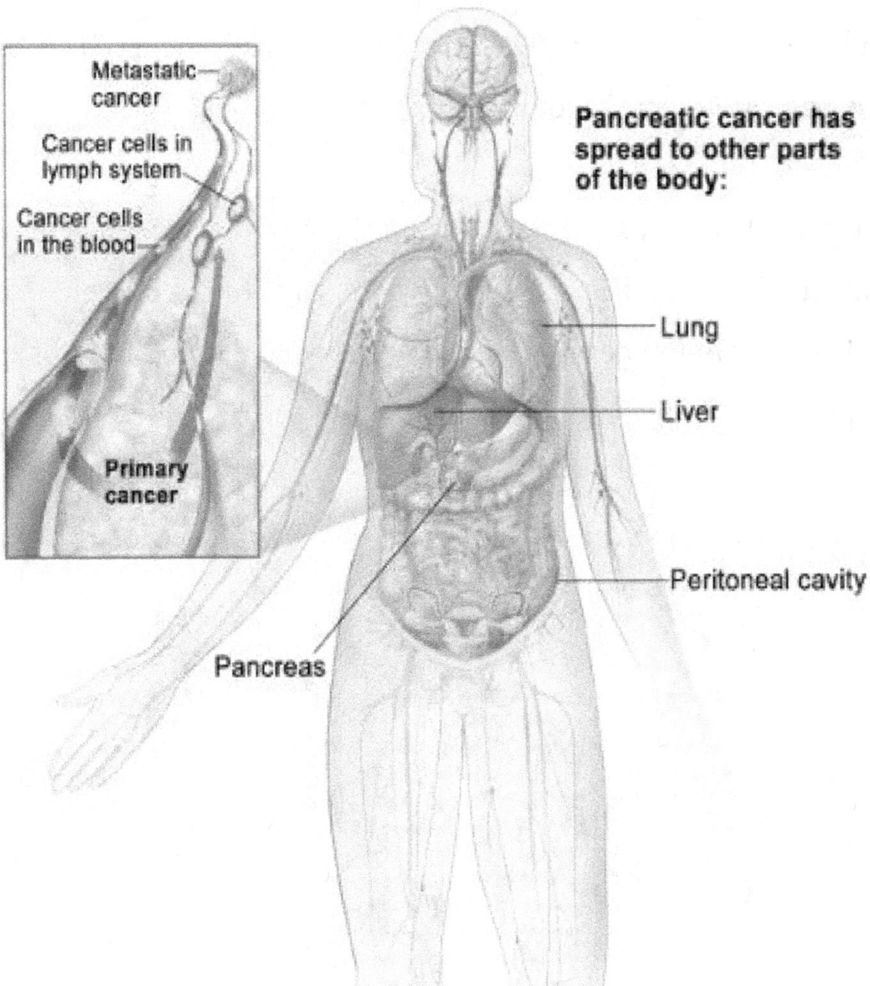

The N stage of pancreatic cancer refers to the presence of lymph nodes that contain cancer cells. N0 means no cancer cells in the lymph nodes, while N1 indicates that cancer cells are present.

The M stage of pancreatic cancer refers to the presence of metastases. M0 indicates that there is no evidence of metastases, while M1 indicates that the cancer has spread to distant organs or tissues.

Once the T, N, and M stages of pancreatic cancer have been determined, they are combined to determine the overall stage of the cancer. **Stage I** pancreatic cancer is confined to the pancreas and has not spread to lymph nodes or distant organs.

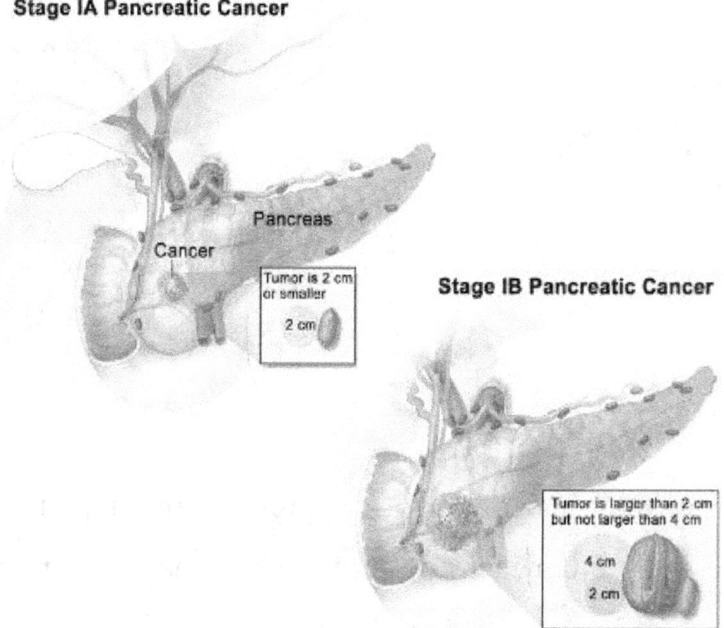

Stage II pancreatic malignant growth has spread to local lymph hubs, yet not to far off organs.

Stage III pancreatic cancer has spread to nearby organs or tissues, but not to distant organs.

Stage IV pancreatic cancer has spread to distant organs or tissues.

Staging pancreatic cancer is important in determining the best course of treatment and prognosis for a patient. Early-stage pancreatic cancer is often treated with surgery, while advanced-stage pancreatic cancer is typically treated with chemotherapy and/or radiation therapy. Patients with early-stage pancreatic cancer often have a better prognosis than those with later-stage pancreatic cancer. Therefore, it is important to accurately stage pancreatic cancer so that the best treatment and prognosis can be determined.

Different Stages of Pancreatic Cancer

1. Localized: This is the earliest stage of pancreatic cancer, and is characterized by the cancer being confined to the pancreas. At this stage, the cancer has not spread to any other parts of the body. An example of localized pancreatic cancer would be an early-stage ductal adenocarcinoma (a common type of pancreatic cancer) that has not spread to any lymph nodes or distant organs.

2. Regional: This stage of pancreatic cancer is characterized by cancer that has spread beyond the pancreas to nearby lymph nodes or the surrounding tissue. An example of regional pancreatic cancer would be a ductal adenocarcinoma that has spread to nearby lymph nodes.

3. Locally Advanced: This is a stage of pancreatic cancer where the tumor has grown large enough to invade and/or damage nearby organs. An example of locally advanced pancreatic cancer would be a ductal adenocarcinoma that has spread to the duodenum (the first part of the small intestine).

4. Metastatic: This is the most advanced stage of pancreatic cancer, and is characterized by the cancer having spread to other parts of the body, such as the liver or the lungs. An example of metastatic pancreatic cancer would be a ductal adenocarcinoma that has spread to the liver.

C. Risk Factors for Pancreatic Cancer

Pancreatic cancer is one of the most serious and deadly forms of cancer. It has been estimated that, in 2020, almost 57,600 people in the United States alone will be diagnosed with pancreatic cancer and over 47,000 will die from the disease. In the United States, pancreatic cancer is the third leading cause of cancer-related death, accounting for more than 7% of all cancer deaths. The risk factors for pancreatic cancer vary, but some of the most common include age, gender, race, family history, lifestyle, and environmental factors.

<u>**Age**</u>: Age is one of the most common risk factors for pancreatic cancer. The incidence of pancreatic cancer increases with age, with the majority of people diagnosed being over the age of 65. It is more common in men than in women, though women are at higher risk after the age of 70.

Gender: Men are at a higher risk of pancreatic cancer than women. In fact, men are twice as likely to develop pancreatic cancer than women, and the incidence rate for men increases with age.

Race: African-Americans have the highest rate of pancreatic cancer in the United States, with an incidence rate of about 1.5 times higher than

Caucasian individuals. Asian Americans, Hispanic Americans, and Native Americans also have higher rates than Caucasians.

Family History: A family history of pancreatic cancer is one of the most significant risk factors for the disease. People with a first-degree relative (parent, sibling, or child) who has had pancreatic cancer have a two- to three-times greater risk of developing the disease than people with no family history.

Lifestyle: Diet is an important risk factor for pancreatic cancer. People who consume a diet high in red and processed meats, as well as foods high in fat, have an increased risk of developing the disease.

Smoking is another lifestyle factor that has been linked to an increased risk of pancreatic cancer. People who smoke have a two- to three-times greater risk of developing the disease than those who do not smoke.

Environmental Factors: Exposure to certain environmental toxins, such as asbestos, can increase the risk of pancreatic cancer. Other environmental factors, such as air pollution, have also been linked to an increased risk of the disease.

Others include;

Diabetes: Diabetes is a metabolic disorder characterized by high levels of glucose in the blood due to a deficiency of insulin production or insulin resistance. Diabetes increases the risk of pancreatic cancer because it causes several changes to the pancreas and its functions. Over time, high levels of glucose can damage the cells in the pancreas and lead to inflammation, leading to the formation of tumors.
 Additionally, people with diabetes tend to have higher levels of insulin in the blood, which can also increase the risk of pancreatic cancer. Long-term diabetes can also lead to the development of metabolic syndrome, which is associated with an increased risk of pancreatic cancer.

Obesity; Obesity is a strong risk factor for pancreatic cancer, as it increases the risk of developing the disease.
Excess body fat has been linked to an increased risk of developing pancreatic cancer, especially in those who are overweight or obese. This is due to the presence of higher levels of certain hormones, such as insulin and estrogen, which are known to stimulate the growth of pancreatic cancer cells. In addition, obesity is associated with an increase in inflammation, which is thought to contribute to the development of pancreatic cancer.

Finally, obesity may increase the risk of pancreatic cancer due to its effects on blood sugar and fat metabolism, which can lead to cell damage.

Exposure to certain chemicals: Exposure to certain chemicals is a risk factor for pancreatic cancer because some chemicals, such as benzene, can cause cellular damage and mutations. Exposure to these chemicals can increase the risk of pancreatic cancer because they can damage the DNA in cells, leading to uncontrolled growth and the development of a tumor. Additionally, some of these chemicals can interfere with the body's natural defenses against cancer, making it more likely that cancer cells can develop and spread. Long-term exposure to these chemicals, either through the workplace or through environmental factors, can increase the risk of pancreatic cancer.

CHAPTER 2

Diagnosing and Treating Pancreatic Cancer

A. Diagnosing Pancreatic Cancer

Diagnosis of pancreatic cancer usually involves a combination of medical imaging, blood tests, and biopsy. It is important to check for other medical conditions that may be causing the symptoms, such as pancreatitis or gallstones, before confirming a diagnosis of pancreatic cancer. The following are some of the most common ways to diagnose pancreatic cancer.

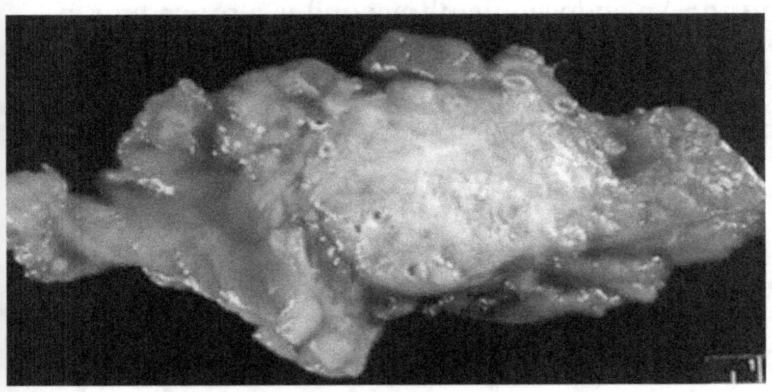

<u>Imaging Tests</u>: Imaging tests such as CT scans, MRI scans, and ultrasound are used to detect tumors and other abnormalities in the pancreas. These tests can also detect enlarged lymph nodes, which may be an indication of cancer. In some cases, a special type of imaging called PET scans may be used to detect the spread of the cancer to other organs.

<u>Blood Tests</u>: Blood tests such as CA19-9, CEA, and CA125 may be used to detect elevated levels of certain proteins and other markers that can indicate the presence of cancer.

<u>Biopsy:</u> A biopsy is the most accurate way to diagnose pancreatic cancer. During a biopsy, a small piece of tissue is removed from the pancreas and examined under a microscope. This will allow doctors to determine if the cells are cancerous or not.

<u>Endoscopic Ultrasound</u>: An endoscopic ultrasound is a procedure in which a thin, flexible tube with an ultrasound probe is inserted through the mouth and into the stomach and intestines. This allows the doctor to view the pancreas and take tissue samples for further testing.

<u>Endoscopic Retrograde Cholangiopancreatography (ERCP)</u>: This procedure uses a combination of X-rays and an endoscope to examine the pancreas, bile ducts, and gallbladder. A special dye is used to make the organs more visible and a biopsy may be taken during the procedure.

<u>Laparoscopy</u>: During a laparoscopy, a thin, flexible tube with a small camera is inserted through a small incision in the abdomen. This allows the doctor to view the pancreas and take tissue samples for further testing.

B. Treating Pancreatic Cancer

Pancreatic cancer is one of the deadliest forms of cancer, with a 5-year survival rate of just 8%. It is an aggressive disease that is difficult to detect in its early stages and is often diagnosed at a late stage when cancer has already spread to other organs. Treatment options for pancreatic cancer include surgery, chemotherapy, radiation therapy, targeted therapy, and immunotherapy.

Surgery:

Surgery is one of the most common treatments for pancreatic cancer. It involves the removal of the tumor, surrounding tissue, and lymph nodes to try to reduce the risk of the cancer spreading.

Examples of surgeries used to treat pancreatic cancer include:

- ***Whipple procedure***: This procedure involves the removal of the head of the pancreas, the gallbladder, and part of the small intestine.

- ***Distal pancreatectomy:*** This procedure involves the removal of the tail and body of the pancreas.

- ***Total pancreatectomy***: This procedure involves the removal of the entire pancreas, gallbladder, and spleen.

- ***Pancreaticoduodenectomy:*** This procedure involves the removal of the head of the pancreas, the gallbladder, part of the small intestine, and sometimes part of the stomach.

Surgery is often used in combination with other treatments such as chemotherapy, radiation therapy, or immunotherapy. Surgery can help to reduce the risk of the cancer spreading, but it is not always successful. It is important to discuss the risks and benefits of surgery with a doctor before making a decision.

Chemotherapy

Chemotherapy is a treatment for pancreatic cancer that uses drugs to kill cancer cells. It is typically administered intravenously or taken orally as a pill. Chemotherapy works by targeting rapidly dividing cells, including cancer cells, and interfering with their ability to divide and grow.

Examples of chemotherapy drugs used to treat pancreatic cancer include gemcitabine (Gemzar®), 5-fluorouracil (5-FU), capecitabine (Xeloda®), oxaliplatin (Eloxatin®), and irinotecan (Camptosar®). These drugs are usually used in combination with one another, as well as with other treatments such as radiation and surgery.

Chemotherapy can be an effective treatment for pancreatic cancer, but it is not always successful. Side effects may include nausea, vomiting, hair loss, fatigue, and increased risk of infection. Patients should discuss all potential risks and benefits of chemotherapy with their doctor before starting treatment.

Radiation Therapy

Radiation therapy is a type of cancer treatment that uses high-energy radiation to kill cancer cells or keep them from growing and dividing. When used to treat pancreatic cancer, radiation therapy can be used to shrink a tumor and relieve symptoms such as pain. Surgery and chemotherapy, for example, can be used in conjunction with radiation therapy.

Radiation therapy for pancreatic cancer is usually delivered through external beam radiation, which is radiation that is delivered from a machine outside the body. The radiation is aimed directly at the tumor and the surrounding area. Radiation may also be delivered through internal radiation, which is radiation that is placed inside the body near the tumor. Internal radiation is usually delivered through tiny radioactive seeds.

Radiation therapy is often used to treat pancreatic cancer when it is not possible to surgically remove the tumor. Radiation therapy can also be used in combination with chemotherapy to shrink the tumor and reduce the risk of cancer coming back. After surgery, radiation therapy may be used to kill any cancer cells that remain.

Targeted therapy

Targeted therapy is a type of cancer treatment that uses drugs or other substances to identify and attack specific types of cancer cells without harming normal cells. It is a type of systemic therapy, meaning it can affect cells throughout the body. Targeted therapy is used to treat a variety of cancers, including pancreatic cancer.

Examples of targeted therapies used to treat pancreatic cancer include drugs such as gemcitabine, erlotinib, and capecitabine, as well as immunotherapies such as nivolumab and ipilimumab. These therapies work by blocking, inhibiting, or suppressing specific proteins that act as markers for cancer cells, allowing them to be targeted and destroyed.

Immunotherapy

Immunotherapy is an emerging treatment for pancreatic cancer that uses the body's immune system to fight the cancer. Immunotherapy works by either helping the body's immune system recognize and attack cancer cells or by helping the body produce substances that target and destroy cancer cells. Examples of immunotherapies used to treat pancreatic cancer include:

• <u>Checkpoint inhibitors</u>: These drugs block checkpoints that cancer cells use to hide from the immune system. Examples include Yervoy (ipilimumab) and Keytruda (pembrolizumab).

• <u>Monoclonal antibodies:</u> On the surface of cancer cells, these medications target specific proteins. Examples include Erbitux (cetuximab) and Cyramza (ramucirumab).

• <u>Vaccines:</u> These drugs stimulate the immune system to attack cancer cells. Examples include CRS-207 and GVAX.

• <u>Oncolytic viruses</u>: These viruses are designed to specifically target and kill cancer cells while leaving healthy cells unharmed. Examples include Imlygic (talimogene laherparepvec) and Pexa-Vec (JX-594).
These are some of the most common treatments for pancreatic cancer. To increase the likelihood of survival, a combination of treatments may be used in some instances.Talking to your doctor about the best course of treatment for you is crucial.

Remember, pancreatic cancer is one of the deadliest forms of cancer and is difficult to detect in its early stages. Surgery, chemotherapy, radiation therapy, targeted therapy, and immunotherapy are all options for treatment. Talking to your doctor about the best course of treatment for you is crucial.

C. Clinical Trials for Pancreatic Cancer

Clinical trials are research studies that evaluate the safety and effectiveness of new treatments for pancreatic cancer. They are conducted to determine if the new treatment can improve the patient's quality of life, extend life expectancy, or reduce the risk of cancer spreading. Clinical trials are the main way that new treatments for pancreatic cancer are developed and tested.

Clinical trials involve giving the patient an experimental drug or treatment and then measuring the results. Results may include changes in symptoms, tumor size, or other measures of the patient's health. The study is carefully designed to ensure that the results are accurate and reliable.

Pancreatic cancer clinical trials are conducted in stages. In the early stages, the drug or treatment is tested on a small group of patients. The goal is to determine if the treatment is safe and effective. If the results are promising, the trial moves to the next stage, which includes a larger group of patients. This allows for more detailed analysis of the results.

In the later stages of the trial, the drug or treatment is tested in a much larger group of patients. This allows the researchers to collect data from a larger population of patients. The results from the later stages are used to determine if the drug or treatment is safe and effective for use in the general population.

Before participating in a clinical trial, patients should speak with their doctor about the risks and benefits of the trial. Clinical trials are overseen by an independent board of experts to ensure the safety of the patients. Patients should also be aware that there is no guarantee that the experimental drug or treatment will work.

Clinical trials are essential in the development of new treatments for pancreatic cancer. By participating in a clinical trial, patients can gain access to new treatments that may improve their quality of life and extend their life expectancy. However, they should also be aware of the risks and potential side effects associated with the trial.

CHAPTER 3

Living with Pancreatic Cancer

A. Adjusting to a New Normal

Adjusting to a new normal life with pancreatic cancer can be difficult and overwhelming. It is important to give yourself time and space to process the diagnosis and adjust to the new situation.

First, it is important to establish a new routine. This may involve changes in diet, exercise, medications, and other health-related activities. Having a routine helps you to stay organized, focused, and on track. Additionally, it relieves anxiety and stress. You may also want to set aside time for self-care to reduce stress and cope with any emotional distress.

Good diets are important for Pancreatic cancer patients:

- Eat a balanced diet that is low in fat, high in fiber and rich in antioxidant foods. Whole grains, lean proteins, a lot of fruits and vegetables, and healthy fats should all be included.

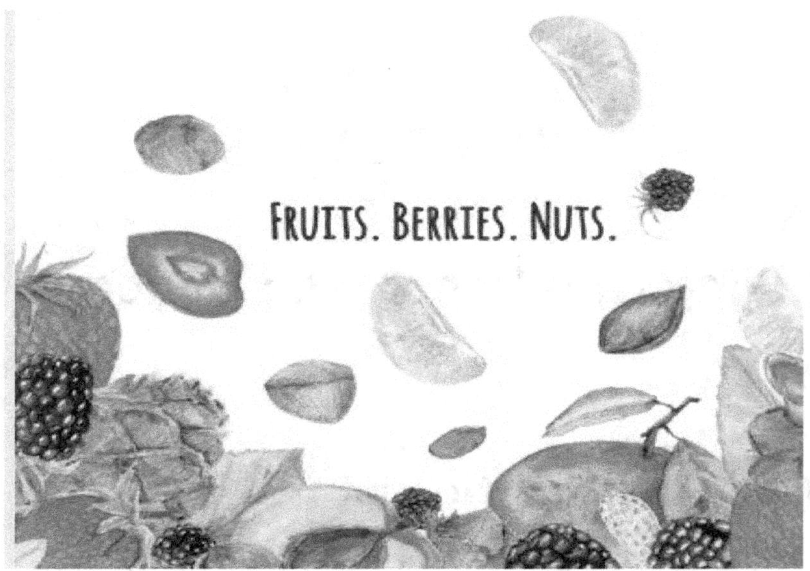

- Avoid processed foods and refined sugars, as they can increase the risk of pancreatic cancer.

- Limit red meat consumption and choose lean proteins such as fish, poultry, eggs, and legumes.

- Avoid fried foods and opt for natural sources of fat, such as nuts, seeds, and avocado.

- Choose low-glycemic index carbohydrates, including whole grains, legumes, and most fruits and vegetables.

- Drink plenty of fluids, particularly water, to stay hydrated and reduce the risk of dehydration.

- Limit alcohol consumption and avoid smoking.

- Exercise regularly to help maintain a healthy weight and improve overall wellbeing.

Second, it's critical to establish a network of support. This could include family, friends, and healthcare professionals. It is important to have someone to talk to who can understand what you are going through. Additionally, having a support system can help you to stay positive, as it can provide encouragement and help you not feel alone.

Third, it is important to stay connected with others. Reaching out to friends and family can provide a sense of comfort and help reduce isolation. Additionally, you can stay connected to the pancreatic cancer community through online support groups and forums. These can give significant data and assets, as well as consistent encouragement.

Finally, it is important to focus on the positive and to set realistic goals. It is important to remember that life does not have to stop after a pancreatic cancer diagnosis. Set small, achievable goals, such as taking a walk around the block or learning a new skill. These goals can help you to focus on the present and to stay motivated.

Adjusting to a new normal with pancreatic cancer can be challenging, but it is possible to live a happy and fulfilling life. By creating a new routine, building a support system, staying connected with others, and setting realistic goals, you can adjust to the new normal.

B. Coping Strategies for Living with Pancreatic Cancer

Coping with pancreatic cancer can be an incredibly difficult and emotional process. It is important to remember that you are not alone in this journey, and there are many strategies that can help you cope.

1. Educate Yourself: It can be helpful to learn as much as you can about pancreatic cancer, including available treatments, side effects, and prognosis. This can help you feel more in control and prepared for the road ahead.

2. Connect with Others: Join a support group or connect with people who are also going through the same experience. It can be comforting to talk to others who understand what you're going through.

3. Stay Positive: Remind yourself that pancreatic cancer is treatable and that many people have been successful in their fight against it. Keeping a positive attitude can help you stay strong and focused.

4. Take Time for Yourself: Make sure you are taking time to rest, relax, and do things that you enjoy. This can help you cope with the anxiety and stress of the situation.

5. Exercise: Exercise can help reduce stress and improve your physical and emotional health.

6. Eat Healthy: Eating a healthy diet can help your body heal and cope with the side effects of cancer treatments.

7. Practice Relaxation Techniques: Meditation, yoga, and deep breathing can help you relax and find peace.

By employing these strategies, you can help yourself cope with the emotional and physical challenges of pancreatic cancer. Remember, you are not alone in this journey, and there are many resources available to help you.

C. Support for Caregivers

Support for caregivers of people living with pancreatic cancer is extremely important. Caregivers can provide physical, emotional, and practical support to the patient. Caregivers may be family members, friends, or even professional medical staff.

Caregivers can help the patient with everyday tasks such as getting dressed, bathing, and eating. They can also help manage medications, attend doctor's appointments, and provide emotional support. Caregivers can also help with activities of daily living, such as grocery shopping and housekeeping.

Support can also be found in health care providers and organizations. Organizations such as the Pancreatic Cancer Action Network, American Cancer Society, and Pancreatic Cancer UK offer resources for patients and caregivers. These organizations provide information about treatments, support groups, and financial assistance.

Caregivers can also seek support and resources from other caregivers. Many online support groups provide a forum for caregivers to connect and share their experiences. These groups can provide a sense of community and understanding that can be helpful during difficult times.

Finally, professional counseling can also be helpful. Counselors can provide support and strategies to cope with the demands of being a caregiver. They can also provide resources and referrals to other services that may be helpful.

CHAPTER 4

Resources for Patients and Families

Pancreatic cancer is a serious and life-threatening disease that can affect both patients and their families. It is important for patients and their families to have access to resources that can help them cope with the diagnosis, treatment, and long-term care. Below are a few resources for patients and families living with pancreatic cancer.

A. Financial and Insurance Assistance

Financial and insurance assistance can be a crucial factor in helping people living with pancreatic cancer. Depending on their individual situation, people with pancreatic cancer may be able to take advantage of a range of financial and insurance assistance programs, including:

Medicare: Medicare is the federal health insurance program that provides coverage for people who are 65 and older, as well as those with certain disabilities. People with pancreatic cancer may be able to receive coverage for medical treatments, doctor visits, and hospital stays.

Medicaid: Medicaid is a state-run program that provides health coverage for people with low incomes. People with pancreatic cancer may be eligible for coverage for medical treatments, doctor visits, and hospital stays.

Cancer Insurance: Cancer insurance is a type of insurance policy designed to provide financial assistance to people with cancer. Depending on the policy, it may cover medical bills, lost wages, and other costs associated with cancer treatment.

Financial Assistance Programs: Many organizations provide financial assistance to people with pancreatic cancer. These programs may provide funds to help cover medical bills, transportation costs, and other expenses associated with pancreatic cancer care.

Charitable Organizations: There are numerous charitable organizations that provide financial assistance to people.

B. Organizations and Support Groups

Organizations:

Pancreatic Cancer Action Network (PanCAN): PanCAN is a national organization dedicated to fighting pancreatic cancer through research, patient services, advocacy, and community engagement. They provide education, support, and research funding for those affected by pancreatic cancer.

Pancreatic Cancer UK: This organization provides support and information for people living with pancreatic cancer. They offer online support groups, practical advice on managing the disease, and advocacy efforts to increase awareness and improve access to treatments.

Support Groups:

Pancreatic Cancer Support Group: This online support group offers a safe space for individuals to share their experiences, ask questions, and find support from fellow patients and caregivers.

Pancreatic Cancer Survivors: This support group provides a platform for those living with pancreatic cancer to connect and share their stories, tips, and experiences. They also provide information about medical treatments, clinical trials, and other resources.

Pancreatic Cancer Action Network Survivors Network: This network provides peer-to-peer support for individuals living with pancreatic cancer. They provide a variety of programs, such as webinars, support groups, and a community forum.

C. Other Resources

1. Pancreatic Cancer Action Network: https://www.pancan.org/

2. American Cancer Society: https://www.cancer.org/cancer/pancreatic-cancer.html

3. Pancreatic Cancer UK: https://www.pancreaticcancer.org.uk/

4. National Pancreas Foundation: https://www.pancreasfoundation.org/

5. Pancreatic Cancer Research Fund: http://www.pcrf.org/

6. Pancreatic Cancer Canada: https://www.pancreaticcancercanada.ca/

7. Pancreatic Cancer Action: http://www.pancreaticcanceraction.org/

8. Pancreatic Cancer Research Institute:
http://www.pancreaticcancerresearch.org/

9. Pancreatic Cancer Research Fund Alliance: http://www.pcrf-alliance.org/

10. Cancer Research Institute:
https://www.cancerresearch.org/pancreatic-cancer

CONCLUSION

Living with pancreatic cancer is a difficult journey for those afflicted, their families, and the medical professionals who care for them. Despite the difficult journey, there is hope for those battling the disease. The most important thing to remember is that pancreatic cancer is treatable, and with the right care and support, it can be managed.

Although pancreatic cancer is a serious and potentially life-threatening disease, it is also one that can be managed and treated. With the right medical care and support, people living with the disease can maintain a good quality of life. The process can be arduous, but it is possible to live with pancreatic cancer and make the best of the situation.

Living with pancreatic cancer can be challenging and it is important to stay positive, seek support, and take care of your health. With a strong support system and proper medical care, those living with pancreatic cancer can manage the disease and live a full and meaningful life.